SELF-EXAMINATION

By

V.K.Grover

DISCLAIMER AND/OR LEGAL NOTICES

This book is the outcome of my study of **alternative medicines** for last more than 20 years. Self-Diagnosis of diseases is based on my study and observations of different parts of body.

It is now a well-known fact that many diseases can be initially diagnosed by standing before the mirror and closely watching face, tongue, eyes, ears and nails. Pressing the hand, feet and ears at all points and observing if there is any abnormality like soft or hard points on the same can not only indicate the diseased part/likely diseased part of the body but repeatedly pressing these points can even cure the disease. This method has been used by Chinese since centuries and is known as Reflexology. Acupressure/ acupuncture have been now acknowledged through the world for cure. I have tried to give these methods in brief in this book.

My efforts through this book are to let the readers know the limitless values of alternative medicine. I have observed that these simple and cheap methods of diagnosis and cure can go a long way for treatment of diseases.

The information within this book is intended as reference materials only and not as medical or professional advice. Information contained herein is intended to give you the tools to make informed decisions about your lifestyle and health. It should not be used as a substitute for any treatment that has been prescribed or recommended by your doctor. The information presented herein represents the views of the author.

Thanks

I am grateful to God who inspired me to write this book.

I am also thankful to my wife and children and friends for their love and support, without which it would not have been possible to write this book.

Contents

Chapter 1

Introduction

Before visiting doctor for diagnosis it is important that you scan your own body for possible causes of disease. You should stand before a mirror and view your face, tongue, nails, and eyes and see their colour and any other abnormalities as it will give you a broad spectrum of your problem. You should also press each and every point of your hand, any hard, or soft point will disclose the part of your affected body as each part of the hand is connected to specific part of your body. This method of hand checking is known as reflexology and is widely used in china. Chinese/ Ayurvedic testing of pulses also shows you the affected part of body.

There are many methods of self/natural diagnosis. Nails, Tongue, Eyes, Pulses (note plural), and Ear can be used as indicators for diagnosing of diseases. These methods are being widely used through centuries in countries like China and India. Ears resemble inverted fetus and have about 130 points that are connected to various body parts .In India and China people wear ornaments in their ears and nose. Besides the ornamental value it has also curative action. I myself got pin inserted from acupuncturist as treatment for anxiety. Acupuncturing of certain points of ears has been shown for stopping alcoholism and smoking.

Acupressure/acupuncture is widely used throughout the world now for diagnosis and cure. It has been recognized as alternative therapy even by WHO (World Health Organisation).

Even holistic methods of treatment like Reiki can help diagnosis and cure.

This book deals with most of these extraordinary methods of diagnosis and can help readers in their pursuit for healthy life.

Chapter 2

Health Diagnose Through Nails

Nails mirror Health.

Nails are the beautiful part of our body. . Nails also support fashion style. Women like to modify the nails. Sometimes they like give it a color. Besides showing the beauty, nails work as a stethoscope for human health.

Your toenails and fingernails protect the tissues of your toes and fingers as they are the hardest part of body. They are made up of layers of a hardened sulphur rich protein called keratin, which is also in your hair and skin. Your nails' health can be a clue to your overall health. Healthy nails are usually smooth and consistent in colour. Specific types of nail discoloration and changes in growth rate can signal various lung, heart, kidney and liver diseases, as well as diabetes and anaemia. White spots and vertical ridges are harmless. Change of colour on your nails can be a sign you have a disease.

To know the overall health of your body, try to massage each fingernail. If the nail becomes red when pressed, it means you have good blood circulation and have good organs.

Spots on nails generally indicate some deficiency of minerals such as calcium or zinc. A line across all the nails indicates you have had a fever *or* chronic inflammation of some kind during the last four months (the time it takes a nail to grow from bottom to top). The position of the line enables you to calculate when the condition occurred (see diagram b). If such lines appear repeatedly there is something wrong. Check your nails against the diagrams given below. Colour of nails is also indicative of health/disease

A solid white line that travels horizontally across the nail is a sign of arsenic poisoning.

Fingernails also send many other messages. For example, kidney disease can cause the far end of the nails to turn reddish or brownish. Heart and lung problems can cause fingertips to become bulbous – which is called clubbing. If this happens quickly and painfully, it may point to lung cancer. So pay attention to your nails.

"People should watch their nails, if they become painful, if they change in colour or there are marks on the nails, they should get in touch with their medical provider and see if it means anything internally."

Nail problems that sometimes require treatment include bacterial and fungal infections, ingrown nails, tumours and warts. Keeping nails clean, dry and trimmed can help you avoid some problems. Do not remove the cuticle, which can cause infection.

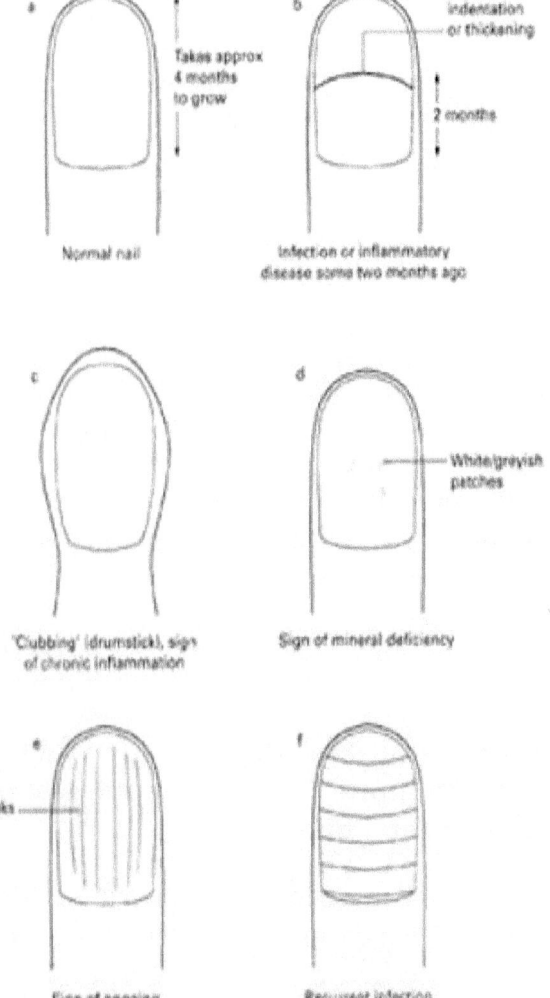

a
Takes approx
4 months
to grow

Normal nail

b
Horizontal
indentation
or thickening

2 months

Infection or inflammatory
disease some two months ago

c
'Clubbing' (drumstick), sign
of chronic inflammation

d
White/greyish
patches

Sign of mineral deficiency

e
Streaks

Sign of ongoing
chronic diseases

f
Recurrent infection
or inflammation

The main function of nails is to protect the soft fingertip. While at the base of the cuticle protects the nail from the discharges. Generally nails has reddish colour as the skin under the nails has many capillaries and are rich in blood supply. However, various circumstances may cause changes in colour and texture of nails, such as:

- Injuries caused by the collapse of a heavy object on the finger nails. These injuries can cause the nails appear blackish color.

- Nail color changes can also be caused by fungal infections.

- Injuries can also cause the formation of spots or white lines on nails.

Here are some nail colours that is a sign of a disease:

- Base of the nail is blue: It is indicated that blood circulation is not maximum and it's a symptom of heart disease.

- Half of the nail tip pink or brown color while the epidermis in white color indicates kidney disease.

- Nail looks dull and there are horizontal wrinkles: indicate malnutrition, the symptoms of measles, chicken pox and mumps.

- Red layer longitudinal on the nails: indicate bleeding in the capillaries, if there is a double line it indicates the symptoms of high blood pressure (hypertension).

- Yellowish of nail color: indicates respiratory diseases like chronic bronchitis.

- Blackish-colored nails: may indicate skin cancer, because it must always be examined to determine whether it is a melanoma (skin cancer).

- Circle crescent in the middle fingernail pink: indicates a person prone to anxiety, susceptible to interference in the internal organs, cannot sleep soundly, frequent headaches.

- Circle crescent on fore finger nails is pink: indicate the weak of intestines and stomach.

- Circle crescent on the ring finger nail pink : indicates the menstruation comes is abnormal

- Circle crescent on the little finger nails pink: indicates a weak of heart condition.

Nail abnormalities are problems with the colour, shape, texture, or thickness of the fingernails or toenails.

Just like the skin, the fingernails tell a lot about your health.

- Beau's lines are depressions across the fingernail. These lines can occur after illness, injury to the nail, and when you are malnourished.

- Brittle nails are often a normal result of aging. However, they also may be due to certain diseases and conditions.

- Koilonychias is an abnormal shape of the fingernail. The nail has raised ridges and is thin and curved inward. This disorder is associated with iron deficiency and anemia.

- Leukonychia is white streaks or spots on the nails.

- Pitting is the presence of small depressions on the nail surface. Sometimes the nail is also crumbling. The nail can become loose and sometimes falls off.

- Ridges are tiny, raised lines that develop across or up and down the nail.

Causes

Injury:

- Crushing the base of the nail or the nail bed may cause a permanent deformity.

- Chronic picking or rubbing of the skin behind the nail can cause a washboard nail.

- Long-term exposure to moisture or nail polish can cause nails to peel and become brittle.

- Fungus or yeast cause changes in the color, texture, and shape of the nails.

- Bacterial infection may cause a change in nail color or painful areas of infection under the nail or in the surrounding skin. Severe infections may cause nail loss.

- Viral warts may cause a change in the shape of the nail or ingrown skin under the nail.

- Certain infections (especially of the heart valve) may cause red streaks in the nail bed.

Diseases:

- Disorders that affect the amount of oxygen in the blood (such as abnormal heart anatomy and lung diseases including cancer or infection) may cause clubbing.

- Kidney disease can cause a build-up of nitrogen waste products in the blood, which can damage nails.

- Liver disease can damage nails.

- Thyroid diseases such as **hyperthyroidism** or **hypothyroidism** may cause brittle nails or splitting of the nail bed from the nail plate (onycholysis).

- Severe illness or surgery may cause horizontal depressions in the nails (Beau's lines).

- Psoriasis may cause pitting, splitting of the nail plate from the nail bed, and chronic destruction of the nail plate (nail dystrophy).

- Other conditions that can affect the appearance of the nails include systemic amyloidosis, malnutrition, vitamin deficiency, and lichenplanus.

- Skin cancers near the nail and fingertip can distort the nail. Subungal melanoma is a potentially deadly cancer that will normally appear as a dark streak down the length of the nail.

- Darkening of the cuticle associated with a pigmented streak may a sign of an aggressive melanoma.

Poisons:

- Arsenic poisoning may cause white lines and horizontal ridges.

- Silver intake can cause a blue nail.

Medications:

- Certain antibiotics can cause lifting of the nail from the nail bed.

- Chemotherapy medicines can affect nail growth.

Normal aging affects the growth and development of the nails.

When to Contact a Medical Professional

Call your health care provider if you have:

- A new or widening dark streak in the nail

- Blue nails

- Clubbed nails

- Distorted nails

- Horizontal ridges

- Pale nails

- White lines

- White color under the nails

If you have splinter haemorrhages, see the doctor immediately.

Prevention

- Do not bite, pick, or tear at your nails (in severe cases, some people may need psychological help or encouragement to stop these behaviors).

- Keep hangnails clipped.

- Wear shoes that don't squeeze the toes together, and always cut the nails straight across along the top.

- To prevent brittle nails, keep the nails short and avoid nail polish. Use an emollient (skin softening) cream after washing or bathing.

Using the vitamin biotin and clear nail polish that contains protein can help strengthen your nails

Images

Nail infection, candidal

Koilonychia

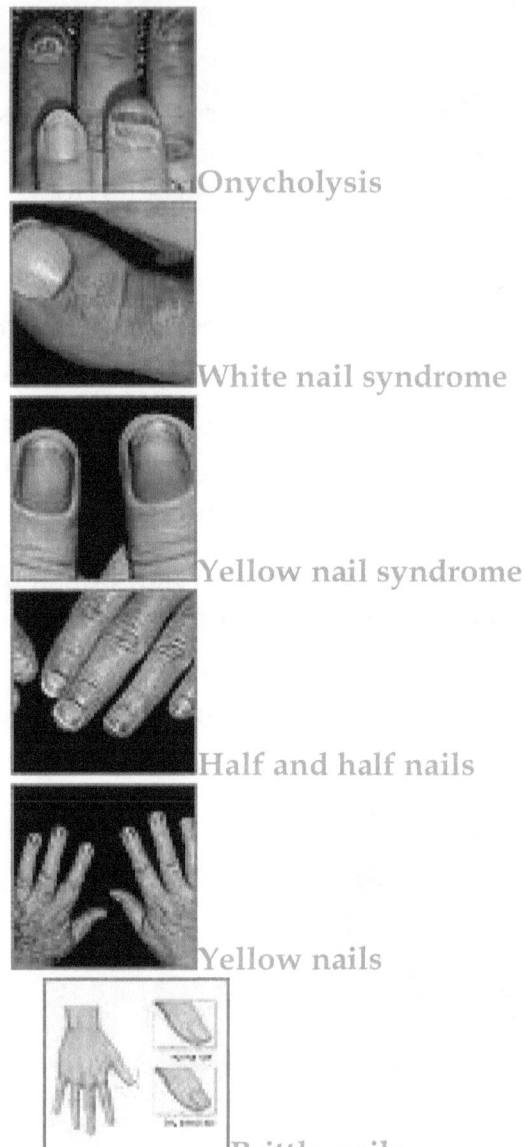

Onycholysis

White nail syndrome

Yellow nail syndrome

Half and half nails

Yellow nails

Brittle nails

Nutritional deficiencies

Vitamin A and calcium deficiencies- dry brittle nails.
Vitamin B deficiency - horizontal and vertical ridges that break easily.
Vitamin B12 deficiency- dry, darkened nails with rounded and curved nail ends.
Protein deficiency- white bands

Ayurvedic analysis:

Nails and body constitution

Ayurveda considers nails as the waste product of the bones.

Dry, crooked, rough nails that break easily indicate a predominance of the Vata constitution.

Soft, pink, tender nails that are easily bent are indication of a Pitta constitution.

Thick, strong, soft and shiny nails indicate a Kapha constitution.

Nails and disease as per Ayurvedic analysis

Longitudinal lines: indicate inability of the digestive system to absorb food properly.
Transverse grooves: may indicate the presence of long-standing illness or malnutrition.
Yellow nails: alert us to liver problems or jaundice.
Blue nails: indicate a weak heart.
Redness: shows an excess of red blood cells.

Homeopathy and nails

The appearance and colour of nails not only reflects the status of our health but can give valuable information about the underlying disease condition and as a homeopath, it can also help us in selecting the most appropriate homeopathic remedy. The following analysis by Dr. Gabrielle Traub gives us an insight into the various states of our nails, their underlying pathology and also the most appropriate homeopathic remedies.

Lines and indentations:

Ridges can signify a possible infection such as the flu.

Beau's lines

Transverse depressions occurs when growth at the nail root (matrix) is interrupted by any severe acute illness e.g. heart attack, measles, pneumonia, or fever. These lines emerge from under the nail folds weeks later, and allow us to estimate when the patient was sick.

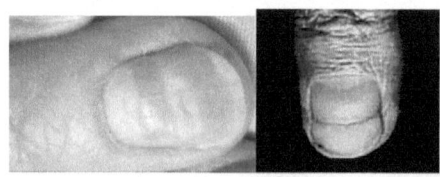

Remedies: **THUJA, GRAPHITES, CALC-FLOUR, SYPH**.

HANDS; NAILS, FINGERS, GENERAL; GROW, NAILS, DO NOT: ANT-C., CALCAREA CARB., SIL.

Medicines: syph (syphilinium), ant-c (antimonium crud), sil (silicea), rad.br (radium bromantum) ,med (*medorrhinum*), anan(*anantheum*), fl-ac (*fluoric acid*)

Mee's lines are

Transverse white lines that run across the nail following the shape of the nail moon.

Uncommon Causality: after acute/severe illness, Arsenic poisoning.

Thus homeopathic remedy= ARS ALB

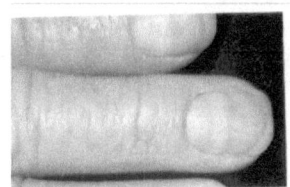

(Lengthwise grooves or ridges) – may indicate a kidney disorder (kidney failure); associated with ageing; iron deficiency (Anaemia). May indicate a tendency to develop arthritis

NAILS; ROUGHNESS FINGERNAILS; RIDGES, LONGITUDINAL: *fl-ac.*

NAILS; ROUGHNESS FINGERNAILS; RIBBED: *thuja.*

NAILS; CORRUGATED: ARS-CALC., CALC-F., FL-AC., MED., PH-AC., SABAD., SEL., SILICEA., THUJA.

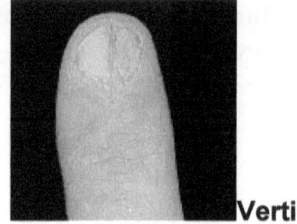
Vertical ridges

Nails shape

Clubbing of the fingers

Fingertips widen and become round. Nails curve around your fingertips, more convex. Proximal nail fold feels spongy caused by enlargement in connective tissue as compensation for a chronic lack of oxygen. e.g. severe emphysema Lung disease is present in 80 percent of people who have clubbed fingers. It may also appear in chronic infections especially abscesses, lung cancer, chronic lung (chronic bronchitis, emphysema) and heart disease, longstanding TB, congenital heart disease, cyanotic, primary biliary cirrhosis.

Medicine: nit-ac., tub.

CURVED FINGERNAILS; CONSUMPTION, IN: MED., TUB.

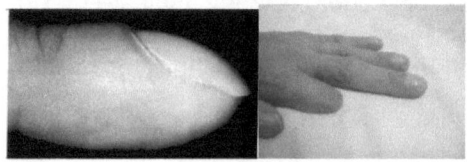

Pitting

Small pits or depressions - Most common nail problem seen in 25 percent to 50 percent of people with psoriasis.

EXTREMITIES; NAILS; HOLES IN: *ars.*

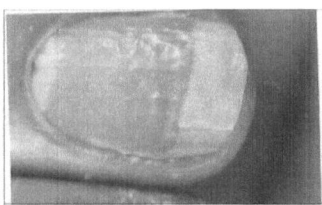

Psoriasis – pitting, onycholysis, thickening, circumscribed yellowish tan discoloration "oil spot" lesion.

Spoon nails

Soft nails that look scooped out. Depression is usually large enough to hold a drop of liquid. Often indicates iron deficiency anaemia.

EXTREMITIES; NAILS; COMPLAINTS OF; DEPRESSED:

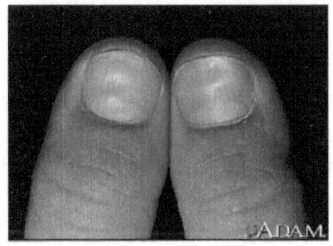

Onycholysis

Lifting of the nail from the nail bed. Causes: trauma, psoriasis, drug reactions, bacterial/fungal infection, contact dermatitis from using nail hardeners, thyroid disease, iron deficiency anaemia or syphilis.

medicnes

LOOSENESS FINGERNAILS: *apis., medorrhinum., pyrogen., ustilago,.*

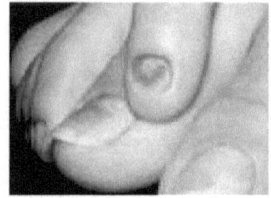

Nail growth

Nail hypertrophy

Thickening of the nail. Either congenital (e.g. Mal de Meleda) or acquired – The nail becomes deformed with claw like appearance.

Causes: Not cutting the nails, trauma, Leprosy, peripheral vascular disorders.

NAILS; HYPERTROPHY: *calc-f., fl-ac., graph., laur.*

NAILS; THICK: ALUM., ANAN., <u>ANT-C.</u>, ARS., BUT-AC., CALC., CALC-FLOUR., CALO., <u>CAUSTICUM.</u>, FALCO-P., FERR., FL-AC., *Graph.*, MERC., PITU-A., POP-C., SABAD., SEC., SEP., *Sil.*, SULPH., <u>UST.</u>, X-RAY

Nail atrophy:

The nail becomes thin, rudimentary and smaller size congenital or acquired. Causes: Lichen planus, Epidermolysis bullosa, Darrier's disease, vascular disturbances, Leprosy.

NAILS; ATROPHIC: *sil.*

NAILS; GROW, DO NOT: *ant-c., pitu-a., rad-br., sil.*

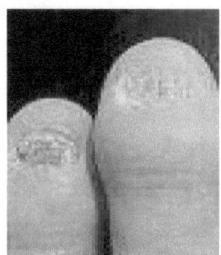

Nail Patella Syndrome

a rare genetic disorder, occurs in 2.2 out of every 100,000 people and causes abnormalities in the bones and nails. Autosomal dominant carried by the ABO blood group.

Nails present as small and concave, longitudinally grooved, abnormally split, pitted, softened, discoloured, or brittle.

Remedies: **THUJA, GRAPHITES, CALC-FLOUR, SYPH**.

H; HANDS; NAILS, FINGERS, GENERAL; GROW, NAILS, DO NOT: **ANT-C., CALCAREA CARB., SIL.**

Medicines: **syph (syphilinium), ant-c (antimonium crud), sil (silicea), rad.br (radium bromantum) ,med (*medorrhinum*), anan(anantheum), fl-ac (fluoric acid)**

Colour of nails is indicative of health/disease

Colour of Nails:

Liver Disease	White
Kidney Disease	Half pink, half white
Lung Disease	Yellow, thick
Diabetes	Yellow, Pink at base

Condition and Nail Appearance:

Nail Bed	Heart Problem	Red
Nail Bed	Anemia	Pale
Discolouration	Fungal Infection	Blue- Green
Discolouration	Bacterial Infection	Yellow, Green or black.

Chapter 3

Tongue

Tongue helps us taste, swallow, and chew. We also use it to speak. Tongue is made up of many muscles. The upper surface contains taste buds. Problems with the tongue include Pain swelling, Changes in color or texture.

Since tongue is highly vascular and contains many important taste receptor cells, it is richly supplied by both the nervous system and circulatory system. It is also constantly nourished or "bathed in" saliva. Saliva is secreted by our salivary glands and controlled by our autonomic nervous system. It contains water, electrolytes, mucus, and enzymes. It serves many functions and can change the appearance of the tongue. *Therefore the tongue is a very sensitive organ and its appearance can change with many physiological changes in the body. By observing the tongue we can see how our whole body is functioning and able to detect imbalances in different systems in our body.*

State of the tongue indicates many problems, especially of digestive system. To know about the body problem, stick out your tongue in front of a mirror and look for the colour, thickness and any other abnormality Ancient Chinese Medicine states that tongue links to various parts on our body and also reflects overall hydration and general circulation of our system. The tongue coating indicates your health conditions or the stage and nature of your disease. A normal tongue should be slightly reddish in color, flexible and coated with a thin, white layer that is neither too moist nor too dry.

Tongue accurately reflects the state of digestive system-from rectum to oesophagus, including the stomach, small intestines, colon (large intestine), pancreas, spleen, liver and gall bladder as shown below.

You don't need lot of tests to find out what part of your digestive tract is in problem. You can diagnosis the whole GI tract and corresponding organ integrity all in one easy view by looking at your tongue.

As a whole the tongue reflects the condition of the digestive system and the organs associated with blood, nutrient assimilation, and excretion. You can also see how 'hot' or how 'cold' your internal organs are. **Therefore it has a high value as a diagnostic tool.**

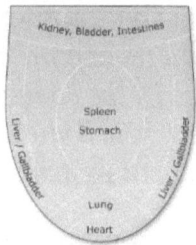

Parts of tongue and connection with body.

When tongue is taken out, the appearance of the tongue is observed in three distinct areas.

The first area is the tongue proper.

We may evaluate the size of the tongue compared to the opening of the mouth or observe any teeth marks on the sides. This may indicate edema or swelling in your body. We may search for any ulcerations or lacerations of the tongue. It may indicate that body is prone or having some form of inflammation. The colour of tongue can give us ideas of the strength of one's health. The normal tongue is pinkish red with a certain shine. When the tongue appears pale, it may be a sign of anaemia or weakened body. When it is red, it may be exhibiting hyperactivity in different systems of the body. When the tongue colour has a tinge of purple, this might be an indication of pain, congestion and blockages in the body. In general, the tongue proper exhibits the strength of your body's own immunity and functioning.

The second area is the tongue coating.

A normal tongue should have a very thin clear coating that exhibits proper enzymatic content and salivary secretions. When the coat becomes thick, it is frequently a sign of imbalance in the digestive system.

When the coat turns thick and cruddy, it is frequently a sign of decreased immune system with Candida (yeast infection) presentation.

When the coat peels, it is frequently a sign of damage or weakening to a certain systems of the body. When the coat turns yellow, it is frequently a sign of infection or inflammation in the body.

The third area is regional analysis.

Different areas of the tongue are represented by the functioning state of different regions of the body. For example, Area A of the tongue represents the functioning of the nervous system and the immune system. Any changes in this area can point to common colds, flu, upper respiratory infections, sleep disorders, and changes in mental state.

Area B of the tongue is represented by the liver and detoxification function of the body. Changes in this region can indicate changing toxicity levels in the body.

Darkening color in this region can mean pain and discomfort in the body. Area C is represented by the functioning of the digestive system and any changes in this area can be an indication of imbalance in the digestion and absorption functions in the body. Area D is represented by the urogenital systems as well as the intestines. Peeling in this region can mean adrenal weakness or chronic low back pains. Thickening of yellow coating in this region can mean either constipation or urinary tract infections. Other changes in this area can indicate problems in the urinary, reproductive and elimination systems.

Specific sections of the tongue mirror the condition of particular parts of the digestive system and the digestion related internal organs.

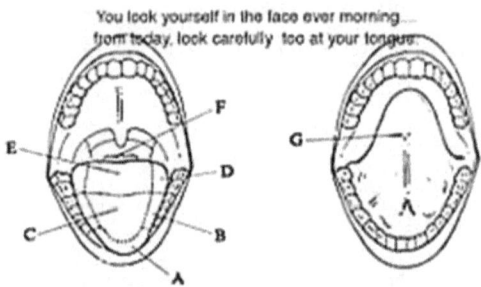

The following correspondences exist in this relationship:

A- The tip area reflects the rectum and the descending colon.

B- The peripheral area reflects the large intestine.

C- The middle region corresponds to the small intestine.

D- The back edge region relates to the liver, gallbladder, duodenum, and pancreas.

E- The near back region corresponds to the stomach.

F- The back region ('the root of the tongue') reflects the oesophagus.

G- The underside of the tongue reflects the quality of blood and lymph circulation in each corresponding area.

But before examination, don't eat foods that may discolor the tongue, such as coffee, beets, vitamin C, and foods made with artificial food coloring.

Some other tongue Tips

- Some disorders don't show up on the tongue.

- Tongue is usually examined for no longer than 15 seconds at a time. If it's extended for longer, the tension may alter the shape or color.

- The tongue should be examined under natural light. Observe your tongue under sufficient lighting and exclude false signs such as a purplish color after sucking blackcurrant lollipop.

Let's start out with the **color of tongue**.

Please pick from one of the following: just focus on the color of the tongue body, not the coating or shape, just the color of the *tongue body*.

[**hint**: if you leave your tongue out for more than 15 seconds it will turn purple. This is normal, just pull your tongue back in, wait a few moments, and then stick it out again. That's the color we want, when it first comes out, not after it turns purple.]

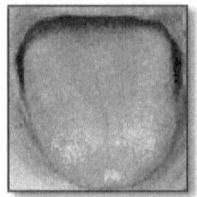 pink tongue body

The pink tongue body color indicates that there is enough energy and is a healthy tongue color. This is a good thing.

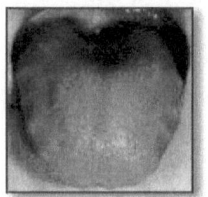 slightly red tongue body

The **(slightly) red tongue body** can be due to a few causes all of which indicate some sort of heat.(may be infection)
A slightly red tongue suggests you're too hot, or not cool enough.
Too much heat means that you've got a fever or some other problematic influence such as an infection or hyper function of one of your organs. Heat can reside in individual organs such as heartburn does in the stomach, or heat can be found everywhere such as you'll find when you have the flu with a fever.

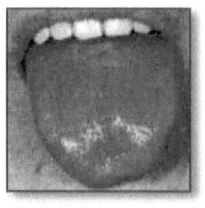 red tongue body

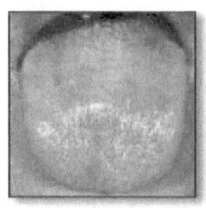 purple tongue body

Purple generally suggests a circulatory issue.
When blood doesn't move well, it isn't properly oxygenated and loses its red color in favor of the blue/purple hues.
However in the wake of a **high fever**, the tongue can look red-purple as an expression of dehydration.

When blood doesn't move well, it isn't properly oxygenated and loses its red color in favor of the blue/purple hues. Red means heat or damage to cooling body fluids. In this case, the problem isn't a circulatory issue but the concentrated color of blood when there is not enough body fluid (or "yin") to thin it out.

However if there is no **high fever** in your immediate past, you may consider one of the following causes for your **purple tongue:**

In general, **Blood stagnation** can give rise to pains that are sharp and fixed in location or lumpy tissues (or both).

This would include angina (chest pains), menstrual cramps, endometriosis, erectile dysfunction, benign or malignant tumors, fibrocystic tissue of the breast or uterus, etc. Erectile dysfunction may also be due to blood stagnation though there's no specific pain or lumps happening, just a deficient circulatory function.

Because "qi leads the Blood", **a stagnation of qi-energy can lead to Blood stagnation**. You can think of qi stagnation as stress-induced neurological issues. These problems can ultimately affect the circulatory system as well. This qi stagnation produces a little heat which can give the tongue some red hue, so it isn't unusual for **Blood stagnation due to qi stagnation** to present with a red-purple colored tongue body.

Internal cold in the abdomen can produce some very deep sharp pains. Internal cold is known to cause one to double over in pain. Cold has a contracting quality to it that causes muscle spasms and severe pains. This purple tongue will actually appear blue-purple since blue is the color of cold.

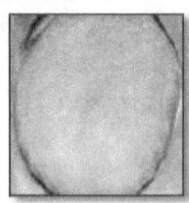 pale or white tongue body

This tongue body indicates a yang-warmth **deficiency** or Blood **deficiency**.

Yang deficiency is a lack of warmth in the body. Your physician may call this a hypothyroid condition or other metabolic deficiency. Symptoms include cold hands and feet, diarrhea, frequent urination, impotence, lack of libido, and fatigue. Since heat rises and "yang" generally rules "up" (while "yin" rules "down") a **yang deficiency** can result in the lack of qi energy and Blood from rising up to nourish (and color) the tongue.

Blood deficiency may or may not be synonymous with "anemia".Symptoms associated with **Blood deficiency** include dry eyes, dry and itchy skin, brittle nails, dizziness, insomnia, irregular periods or lack of periods, and tremors. When the body lacks Blood, the tongue appears pale because Blood is red. Chinese medicine can be very self-evident.

The key difference in appearances between the **yang-warmth deficient** tongue and the **Blood deficient tongue** is that the **yang-warmth deficiency** will be very wet because Yang-warmth is in charge of fluid metabolism in the body. **Blood deficiency** by contrast is much closer to a dehydration condition such that the tongue may appear somewhat dry and withered when observed.

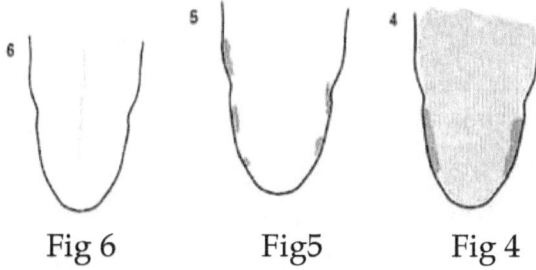

Fig 6   Fig5   Fig 4

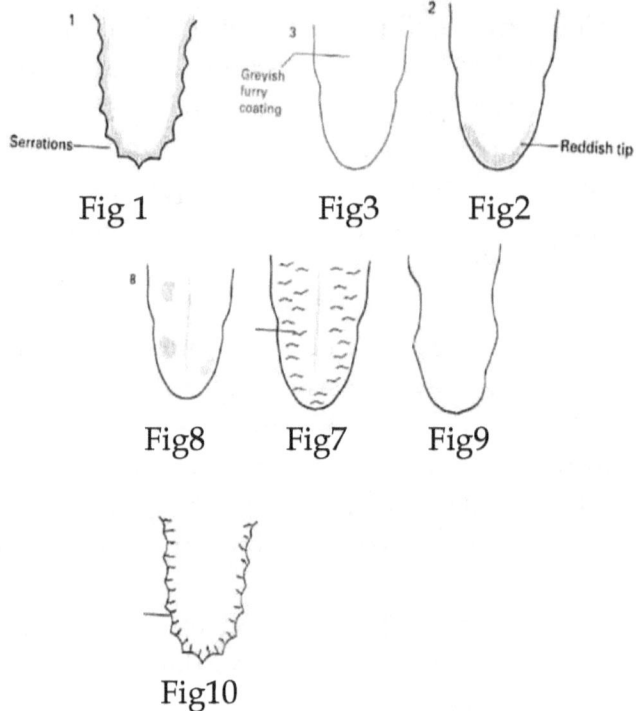

Fig 1 Fig3 Fig2

Fig8 Fig7 Fig9

Fig10

Tongue and diseases

Fig1. Tongue with impressions of teeth- signs of gastritis with acidity.

Fig2. Tongue of a person consuming excess carbohydrates (sweets, chocolate etc).

Fig3. Tongue of a person with constipation or sluggish bowel movements.

Fig4. Tongue with uniform greyish coating and slight reddish irritation on the sides signifies chronic acidity problem (high stomach acid).

Fig5. Tongue showing purple or dark patches indicating chronic anemia (past or current).

Fig6.Tongue showing evidence of 'gut fermentation' or mild yeast overgrowth in the abdomen. Patient may complain of flatulence, cramps etc.

Fig7. Also known as 'geographical tongue'. Indicates signs of liver malfunction, sluggish liver. Could also indicate psoriasis.

Fig8. Ulcerations on the tongue. Shows signs of severe fungal or yeast overgrowth in the abdomen. Deficiency of vitamin B.

Fig9. Severe gastritis or stomach ulcer.

Fig10. Dehydrated tongue (slightly shriveled) with a shiny coating of saliva-signs low water consumption.

Biochemical and tongue

Biochemical treatment is based that all diseases are caused due to deficiency of inorganic salts in the body. The treatment takes into account the condition and colour of tongue to diagnose the disease and deficiency of salt.

Salt	Condition of tongue
Calcarea Fluorica	Cracked appearance of tongue with or without pain. Induration of tongue, hardening after inflammation.
Calcarea Phos	Tongue swollen, numb, stiff, with Pimples on it, white, furred. Bitter taste in morning with headache.
Calcarea	Flabby, resembling a layer of dried clay,

Sulphurica	sour, soapy, acrid taste. Yellow coating at base.
Ferrum Phos	Furred tongue, or clean and red, with headache. Inflammation of tongue with dark red swelling.
Kali Mur	Coating of tongue grayish white, dryish or slimy
Kali Phos	Excessively dry in the morning. White, slimy, brownish like French mustard. Edges of tongue red and sore
Kali Sulphuricum	Coating yellow and slimy, sometimes with whitish edge. Lips, tongue and gums white, taste lost
Magnesium Phos	Generally clean. Coated white with diarrhea, left side sore making eating painful as if scalded.
Natrum Mur	Coating slimy, clear and watery, loss of taste Vesicles on the tip of the tongue, mapped tongue
Natrum Phos	Moist, creamy or golden yellow coating at the back part of tongue. Blisters and sensation of hairs on tip of tongue. Difficult speech.
Natrum Sulphurica	Dirty, brownish green coating or grayish green. Palate very sensitive, better taking cold things. Taste bitter, slimy tongue, Burning blisters on the tip, red tongue.
Silicea	Induration of tongue, ulcer on tongue, sensation of hair on tongue.

Chinese medicine also uses the tongue to interpret health

Zetsu Shin as it is called in Japanese is one of the most important forms of diagnosis used in Chinese medicine. Two main aspects are considered in tongue diagnosis.

First is the structure of the tongue. Is it wide or narrow, Thick or thin, pointed or rounded? Such qualities convey information concerning the individual's basic constitution and overall strengths and weaknesses of body and mind.

Width:

- a wide tongue reflects an overall balanced physical

  and psychological disposition.

- a narrow tongue reflects a lack of physical adaptability

  with pronounced strengths and weaknesses. Mentally,

  thinking may be sharp but tend toward seeing a narrow

  view.

- a very wide tongue reflects a generally loose and

  expanded physical condition and a tendency toward more

  psychological concerns.

Tip:

- a rounded tip reflects a flexible yet firm physical and

  mental condition.

- a pointed tip reflects a tight, perhaps even rigid

physical condition and an aggressive or even offensive mentality.

- a very wide tip reflects an overall weakness of the physical body and a flaccid or even "spaced out" mental condition.

- a divided tip reflects a tendency toward physical and mental imbalances with the possibility of sharp fluctuations in thinking and mood.

Thickness:

- a flat tongue reflects a balanced condition and the ability
to flexibly adapt to circumstances.

- a thin tongue reflects a more mental orientation, with a tendency to be more gentle and easy going.

- a thick tongue reflects a more physical orientation, with the tendency to be assertive or even aggressive.

In comparison to structure, the condition of the tongue is influenced more by daily lifestyle and provides information about an individual's current state of health.

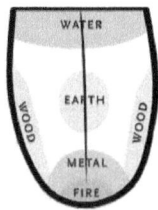

Get in front of the mirror and look at your tongue right now. The tip exhibits the fire element; behind the tongue tip is the metal element; both right and left sides the wood element; in the center towards the back is the earth element; and the very back of your tongue is the water element. Now that you know what element is where, how do you translate what your tongue is telling you?

Signs and symptoms

Here is what you want to see: A normal tongue should be pink, muscular without tooth marking or discoloration, and have a very thin clear coating that exhibits proper salivary secretions. Monitor your evolving health level by noticing color, shape, and coating changes in specific zones.

Tongue Color: When the color becomes deeper — going from pale to scarlet to purple — it means that there is increasing heat in the body. Heat may mean inflammation, infection, or hyperactivity of the organ network.

When the tongue's color becomes lighter — from pink to pale to paper white — it indicates cold, which can mean anemia, pathogenic cold factor, or low energy and function of the corresponding organ to work. Patients with low immune system function, sometimes due to chemotherapy or chronic fatigue syndrome exhibit a pale tongue indicating low energy.

Since tongue is highly vascular and contains many important taste receptor cells, it is richly supplied by both the nervous system and circulatory system. It is also constantly nourished or "bathed in" saliva. Saliva is secreted by our salivary glands and controlled by our autonomic nervous system. It contains water, electrolytes, mucus, and enzymes. It serves many functions and can change the appearance of the tongue. *Therefore the tongue is a very sensitive organ and its appearance can change with many physiological changes in the body.* By observing the tongue we can see how our whole body is functioning and able to detect imbalances in different systems in our body.

- **Lighting**
Sunlight will give the most accurate color of the tongue body and coat. If sunlight is not available, use a second light source such as a small flashlight to compare the tongue color to the original light source.

- **Position**
The tongue should be extended in a relaxed manner, and should not be held out for an extended duration.

- **Food and Drink**
Food and drink, such as coffee, green tea, and candy may alter the color of the tongue coating.

- **Brushed Tongue**
Some patients may brush their tongue to help freshen their breath or as an Ayurvedic practice. Ask the patient not to brush their tongue, at least the day of their TCM

tongue diagnosis.

- **Seasons of the Year**
  In Summer, there may be more Dampness present

  in the tongue coating, leaving it slightly thicker and

  light yellow.
  In Fall or Autumn, the tongue may be thinner with a

  coating that is more dry.
  In Winter, there may also be more moist or damp

  presenting in the tongue.
  In Spring, the tongue should be normal.

- **Time of Day**
  The coating of the tongue usually becomes thinner

  as the day progresses, while the color of the tongue

  body becomes more red and shiny.

- **Patient's Age**
  In the elderly, Qi and Blood Deficiency is more common,

  so the tongue may present with dryness and cracks.
  Infants tend to have white thick coating that is easily

  removed, peeled tongues are also common.
  Overweight patients usually have more Damp

  and/or Phlegm and therefore their tongues may be

  larger and lighter in color.Thin patients tend towards

  redder tongues.

Tongue Body Colour

Indicates the state of Blood, Yin organs, and Ying (Nutritive) Qi.

Normal Tongue Body

- Pink or light red in color

Bluish Purple or Reddish Purple Tongue Body

- Purple can indicate both Heat and Cold conditions.

- A reddish purple tongue indicates Heat and Blood Stagnation.

- A dark reddish purple tongue that is dry usually indicates depleted fluids due to Excess Heat

- A light purple, bluish purple or greenish purple tongue body color can indicate Cold and Blood Stagnation.

Red Tongue Body

- A red tongue body is darker than the normal red, which is pinkish in color. It indicates either Deficient or Excess Heat.

- A red tongue body with a thick yellow coat or swollen buds indicates Excess Heat

- A red tongue body with a bright shiny coat, little coat,

or no coating indicates Deficient Heat.

Red Tip

- Heat in the Heart Zang

Scarlet Tongue Body

- A scarlet tongue that is also peeled or shiny indicates Yin Deficiency, usually of the Heart and/or Lung depending on the area of swelling.

Dark Red Tongue Body

- The red is darker and more crimson in color. This tongue body can indicate internal injury such as trauma (De Da), invasion of external evil in the Ying (Nutritive) and Xue (blood) levels, or it can indicate Blood Stagnation.

- If there are red spots with a thin coat, this usually indicates damage to the Ying or Xue level.

- If the tongue body also has cracks and there is little or no tongue coat, this usually indicates Deficient Heat due to internal injury.

Pale Tongue Body

- Indicates the quality of Blood, reflecting Blood and/or Qi Deficiency or Cold.

- If the tongue body is also moist, tender, and swollen, this can indicate Yang Cold.

- A pale thin tongue body usually indicates Qi and Blood Deficiency.

Green Tongue Body

- A green tongue body usually indicates Excess Yin Cold or the presence of a strong Excess evil with weak Zheng Qi.

The Yang is not properly moving Blood and Fluids and there is Stagnation in the body.

- Internal Wind may also present with a green tongue body.

Tongue Body Shape

The body shape reflects the state of Blood and Ying (Nutritive) Qi, and indicates Excess or Deficiency. Constitution can also affect the shape of the tongue body.

Stiff

- A stiff or rigid tongue is difficult to move (protrude, retract, side to side). This may cause speech abnormalities such as slurring or mumbled speech. A stiff tongue is an indication of Excess, and often one of Internal Wind.

- If a stiff tongue is accompanied by a bluish purple tongue body, this usually indicates potential or impending Wind-Stroke.
- If a stiff tongue is accompanied by a bright red tongue
- body, this usually indicates heat in the Heart and
- Pericardium disturbing the Shen (Spirit).
- If a stiff tongue is accompanied by a thick sticky tongue coating, this usually indicates "Phlegm Misting the Heart".

Flaccid

- The flaccid tongue is the opposite of the stiff tongue. It is weak and lacks strength. It usually indicates Deficiency. When heat has consumed and damaged body fluids, they cannot rise to nourish the tongue. This can indicate Yin Deficiency, Qi Deficiency and/or Blood Deficiency.
- A flaccid tongue that is also pale usually indicates
- Qi and Blood Deficiency.

- A flaccid tongue that is also dark red, dry, and has cracks usually indicates extreme heat injuring fluids.
- A flaccid tongue body with a scarlet tongue body usually indicates Exhaustion of Yin.

Swollen

- This is a very large tongue body and can indicate both Excess and Deficiency.
- A swollen tongue that is also pale can indicate Qi Deficiency
- A swollen tongue that is also bright red and painful can indicate Heart and Spleen Heat. This could also be due to excess alcohol consumption.

Big or Enlarged Tongue

- An enlarged tongue can indicate Phlegm, Damp, or Water Stagnation.
- An enlarged tongue with a pale body and a moist coat may indicate Spleen and Kidney Yang Deficiency
- An enlarged tongue with a red body and a greasy yellow coat may indicate Spleen and Stomach Damp-Heat.

Half the Tongue Is Swollen

- A half swollen tongue may indicate general weakness of the Channels.

Hammer Shaped

- This is where the front half or third of the tongue is enlarged at the sides.

- A hammer shaped tongue usually indicates Spleen, Stomach, and Kidney Deficiency

- This tongue is almost always indicative of a serious condition, and may indicate mental illness.

Local Swelling on One Side

- Localized swelling of tongue with a normal tongue body color indicates Qi Deficiency

- Localized swelling of tongue with a red tongue body color indicates Qi and/or Blood Stagnation

Swollen Sides

- A tongue with swelling in Liver and Gallbladder area usually indicates Rising Liver Yang or Liver Fire.

Swollen Between the Tip and the Central Surface

- This area corresponds to the Lung area and usually presents with a normal or pale tongue body.

- This tongue is usually found in patients with chronic Lung and Spleen Deficiency, which tends toward Damp and Phlegm accumulation.

Swollen Edges

- This tongue may indicate Spleen Qi or yang Deficiency.
- If Spleen Yang is Deficient, the edges will also be wet.

Swollen Tip

- When the very tip of the tongue is swollen, it usually indicates Heart problems.
- If the tongue is also deep red, this may indicate Heart Fire.
- If the tongue is normal in color or pale, this may indicate Heart Qi Deficiency.

Short and Contracted

- When the patient cannot show the entire tongue, it usually indicates a more severe disease.
- If the tongue is also moist and pale, this indicates stagnation of Cold (bluish/purple) in the meridians or Spleen Yang Deficiency.
- If a contracted tongue also has a sticky tongue coating,

this may indicate Turbid-Phlegm blocking the channels.

- If the tongue is also deep red and dry, excessive heat has consumed Body Fluids and stirred up internal Wind.

- A short, swollen, tender, and pale tongue usually indicates Qi and Blood Deficiency.

- A short or small frenum may be inherited and is normal.

Long

- There is difficulty in retracting the tongue.

- This indicates interior Excess Heat, Heart Fire, or Phlegm-Fire Misting the Heart.

- There may be numbness which is associated with

Front Swollen

- Swelling towards the front one-third of the tongue may indicate Phlegm retention in the Lungs.

Thin

- This can indicate that Qi and Blood are deficient and not able to properly nourish and moisturize the tongue. The tongue body will also usually be pale in color with Qi and Blood Deficiency.

- A thin tongue that is also dark red and dry may

indicate Yin Deficient Fire.

Rough or Tender Texture

- A tender tongue that appears smooth, delicate, and is possibly swollen indicates deficiency.

- A rough tongue that appears wrinkled and rough indicates Excess.

Red Spots

Red spots may indicate Heat Toxins in the Blood or Heat Toxins attacking the Heart.

- Red spots can indicate the presence of Damp-Heat in the Xue Level, where the internal organs are accumulating toxins.

- Red spots on the Tip (Lung/Heart area) are usually not severe and may present in the beginning stages of illness.

- Red spots on the entire tongue may indicate a more severe illness.

- Red spots on the sides of the tongue (Liver/Gallbladder area) may also indicate a more severe illness.

- Red spots on the back of the tongue (Kidney area) may indicate the advanced stage or chronic nature of an illness.

White Spots

- White spots are usually due to Spleen and Stomach Qi Deficiency together with excess heat accumulating in the body. In this case, the tongue may also have sores and pus.

Black Spots

- Black spots usually indicate Qi and Blood Stagnation or heat in the Blood.

Deviated Tongue Body

- This is where the tongue tends toward one side of the mouth

- This is due to Wind, either from exterior Pathogenic Wind or internal Wind-Damp patterns.

Moving, Lolling, Wagging, Playful Tongue Body

- This usually indicates heat in the Heart and Spleen channels stirring up internal Wind.

- In children, this may indicate developmental problems.

Teeth Marks on Tongue Body (Scalloped)

- If the tongue body has normal color, this usually indicates Spleen Qi Deficiency

- If there are teeth marks together with a swollen tongue, this may indicate Spleen Yang and/or Qi Deficiency.

- If the tongue is also pale and moist, it is more likely Spleen Yang Deficiency or a Cold-Damp pattern.

Tongue Coating

What does the Tongue Coating Look Like?

Normal tongue coating is thin and white. A pale yellow and Slightly thicker coating at the back of the tongue may also be normal. The tongue coating often indicates the health of the spleen and stomach.

It also provides a good indication of acute illness, such as colds and digestive problems.

The thickness and color of the coating, or a lack of coating, can indicate different issues. When the coat of your tongue becomes thick, it is frequently a sign of imbalance in the digestive system. When the coat turns thick and cruddy, it generally points to decreased immune system with Candida (yeast infection). When the coat turns yellow, it often signals infection or inflammation in the body. A peeling coat is usually a sign of damage or weakening of certain systems of the body.

Tongue coating	May be a sign of
Thick	Excess
Yellow, thick, glossy	Damp heat
Dry, yellow	Excess heat, Deficient yin
Peeled or absent	Heart yin deficiency if it's on the tip of the tongue Kidney yin Heart Yin deficiency if it's all over the tongue or at the back of the tongue and tongue body is red.

Thin Coating

- Normal

- In disease, it indicates the disease is either external or an internal disease that is not severe.

- If the tongue coating changes from thick to thin, this indicates pathogens are moving to the exterior of the body and the disease is waning.

Thick Coating

- A thick coating usually indicates more of an internal
- disease that is more severe.
- It may also indicate that exterior pathogenic factors have penetrated more deeply into the body.
- A thick tongue coating may also indicate retention of food.
- If the tongue coating changes from thin to thick, this indicates pathogens are penetrating deeper into the interior of the body.

Peeled, Mirrored, Shiny, No Coating

- With a mirrored tongue, there is no coating on the tongue. In less severe cases, there may be a partial coating on the tongue.

If the body of the tongue is also red, it usually indicates

- that Stomach Qi and Yin is severely damaged.
- If the tongue body is also light in color, this may

indicate that Qi and Blood of the Spleen and Stomach is damaged and Deficient.

- If the tongue body is also red or dark, Stomach and Kidney Yin is damaged (body fluids dried up) due to heat.

Texture:

- a swollen or enlarged tongue: indicates a Jitsu, or full state.
- A shrivelled or withered-looking tongue: indicates a Kyo, or empty state.

Movement:

- the flexibility of the tongue also reflects the condition of the digestive system. Characteristics to look for include:
  - a flexible, supple, smoothly moving tongue.
  - a stiff, tense, or inflexible tongue.
  - a loose or lolling tongue.
  - a tongue with a pronounced slant to the left or right when it is extended.

Pimples or projections on the tongue's surface indicate the discharge of fat, protein, and sugar. Where in the body this discharge is coming from can be determined by the specific area of the tongue on which it appears. You can find the correlation between the areas of the tongue and

the digestive tract.

Patients with iron deficiency may develop an inflamed,

sore, and swollen tongue. The tongue will appear pale and

smooth due to low levels of hemoglobin in the blood and

the loss of finger-like projections on the surface of the tongue.

Sore and swollen tongue causes problems with chewing,

swallowing and speaking

You can further diagnose underlying problems by analyzing

the regions of your tongue; these show you which organ

network is affected.

1.Tongue tip

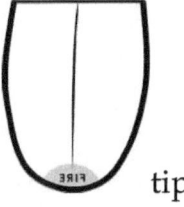 tip

Fire: Cardiovascular System

The fire element zone, which corresponds to the heart-small

intestine network, is located at the tip of the tongue. This includes matters of the heart, both emotions and the physical health. In Chinese medicine, the spirit is said to reside in the heart network. Stress and anxiety will show up as red color and red dots on the tip of the tongue. Increasing heat signs means hyperactivity in the heart network due to stress and tension.

2. Sides of tongue

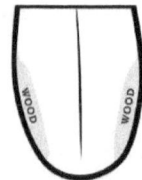

Wood: Liver Network

The sides of your tongue display the wood element. Teeth markings on the sides of the tongue usually mean stagnant energy in the liver network. You may also notice a bluish-green or purplish hue or spots in this zone. Dark spots may indicate more serious problems. On several occasions, purple spots in the wood zone have been

observed in patients that suffer from low energy, discomfort,

distension around the lower ribs, and swelling in the abdomen.

3. Behind the tongue tip

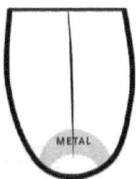

Metal: Respiratory and Immune System
The band-like area across the tongue and just behind the tip

is the metal element zone, which corresponds to the respiratory

and the immune systems. When this area turns reddish, or

when red pin-sized dots occur, it usually means a respiratory

infection is on its way or is settling into the body. Paleness in

the metal zone may reflect a weakened immune system. In

rare fungal infections of the lungs, there may appear a

brownish black coating over this zone, which was the case

with several of patients who suffer from lesions in their lungs.

4.middle of tongue

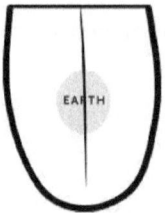

Earth: Digestive System

This area is the earth element zone, and it is related to the stomach-spleen-pancreas network. Problems of the digestive system most often show up here in the center of the tongue. G.E.R.D. — stomach and esophagus acid reflux that keeps many people awake at night — may be seen with redness and a yellowish coating in the center of the tongue. Subtle changes in this area may indicate digestive problems that have not surfaced yet; observe this area and take prophylactic steps if necessary.

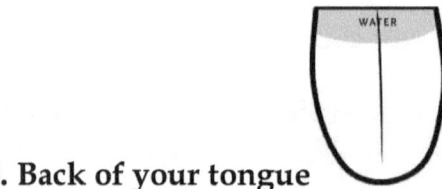

5. Back of your tongue

Water: Kidney-Bladder Network

The back of the tongue reflects many of the body's functions, but is mainly the domain of the water element, or kidney-bladder network, which includes the hormonal system and sexual glands. The two large, elevated papillas on the back of the tongue are a normal part of the taste buds. What you should look for is color and coating. For example, a thick yellow coating at the back-center of the tongue in female patients indicates that they are very likely to get a bladder infection. Drinking 8 to 12 glasses of filtered water a day, taking 5,000 mg of vitamin C, and drinking cranberry juice or taking its extract helps in prevention of bladder infection. Your body alerts you to imbalances in many more ways than just your tongue. Ideally, you should confirm your findings from your tongue with observations from others, such as the eyes, face, and nails.

Chapter 4
Ears

Background

Auriculotherapy applies the principles of reflexology to specific points on the ear. It is a treatment modality where the specific malfunctioning organ or a systemic illness can be treated by application of a laser and/or (transcutaneous electrical nerve stimulation) unit to a correlating part of the external ear.

The point on the ear is located according to a somatotopic map, where each part of the auricle, or external ear, corresponds with a part of the body. The most popular somatotopic map is the "inverted fetus" image, where the organs correspond to the superimposed image of an upside-down person. However, at least four other maps exist to locate and treat maladies of the body. Practitioners may use the somatotopic map to correct imbalances or disease in nearly any part of the body, including chronic health conditions and diseases.

In Auriculotherapy the ear points are used for diagnosis as well as for treatment.

The ear represents the whole anatomical body, but in an upside down position. Dr. Nogier's theory was that the outer

ear e.g the auricle could be compared to an upside-down
 human fetus; the head represented by the lower ear lobe,
the feet at the top of the ear, and the rest of the body
in-between.
This model was first presented to naturopathic practitioners in
France in 1957, then spread to acupuncturists in Germany,
and finally was translated into Chinese. The Chinese adopted
this model in 1958. The earliest use of ear acupuncture points
dates back to ancient China and India. In India people
especially women had been wearing earrings at different
points of ears. This had therapeutic values besides the
ornamental one.
The inverted fetus pattern that is represented on the auricle
is referred to as somatotopic inversion. The word "soma"
means "body" and the word "topic" refers to a topographic
"map." The auricle is a map of the body in an inverted or
down pattern.

This resemblance of body with the fetus and thus to ear is
used for diagnosis and cure of many diseases. Ear has 130
points as shown in the figure below that are used by
acupressurists/acupuncturists to cure the diseases connected
 with various organs.

The points may be detected by inspecting the ear visually
or by pressing the various acupuncture points with a match
stick or a blunt probe and if there is pain in any point, or
any point is hard, it indicates that the corresponding organ
is diseased The acupuncture points may also be detected
using a galvanometer to detect points of reduced electrical
resistance. This is an extremely accurate but time-consuming
form of diagnosis, which can often predict not only existing
illness but also an illness long before it actually occurs.

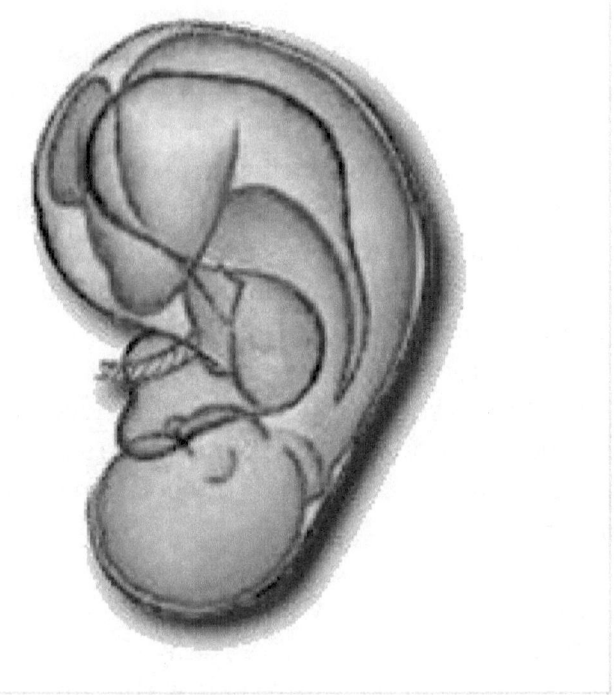

Fig Ear as inverted fetus

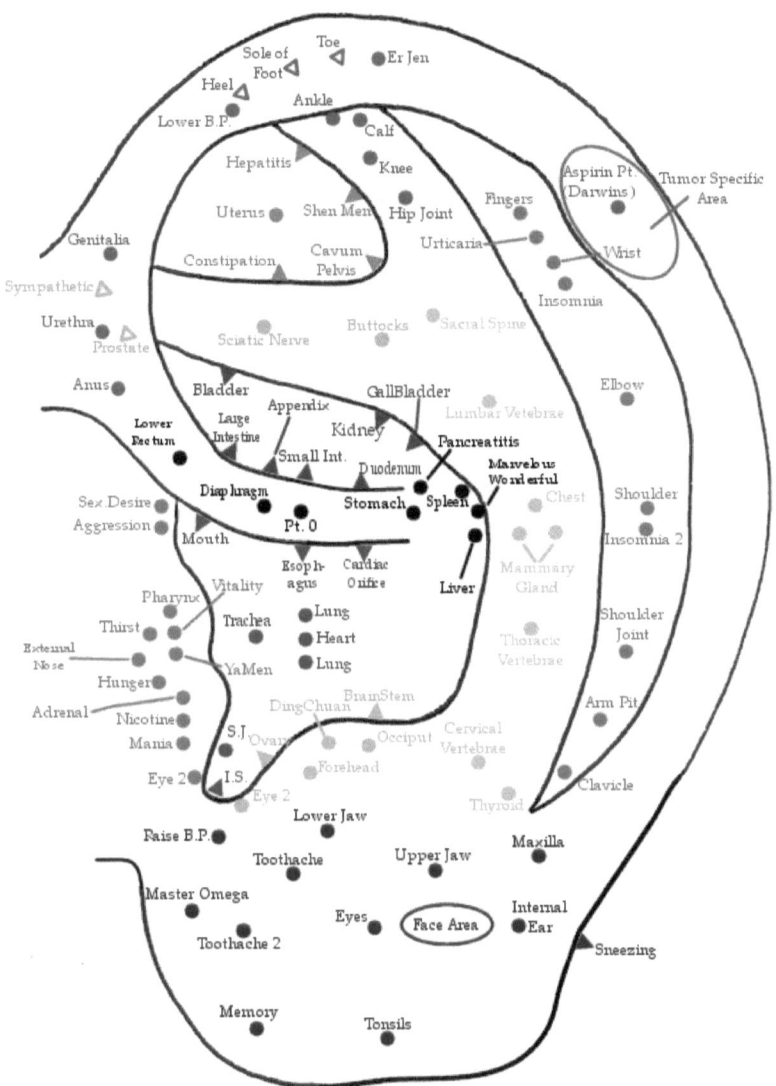

ear points and connected organs

Musculoskeletal points

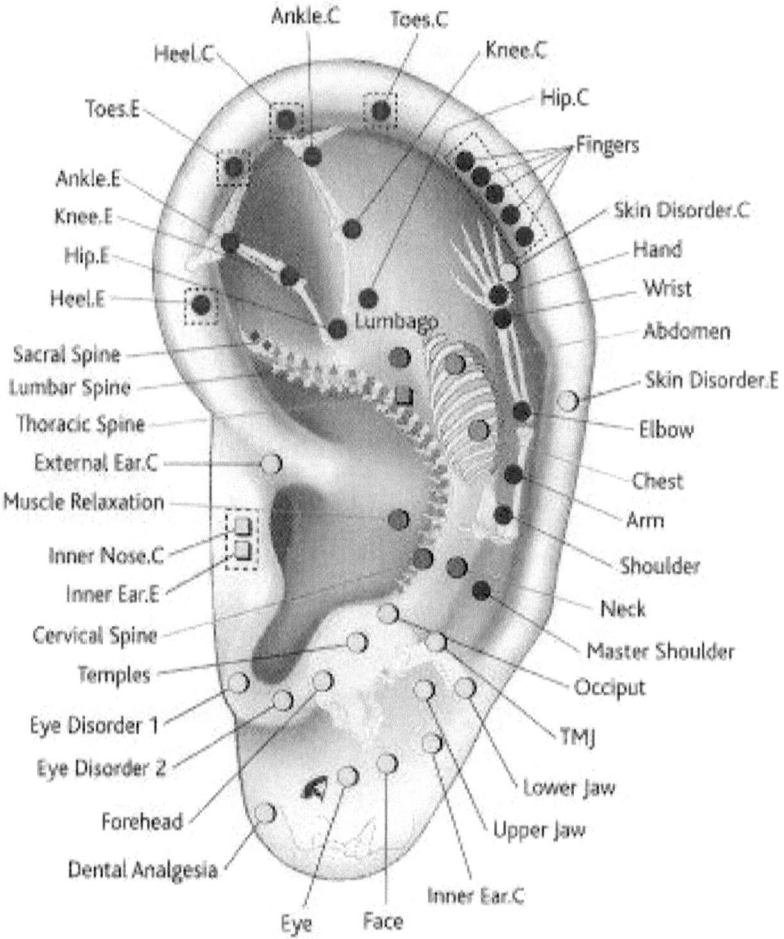

Acupressure points of ear

Other indications of illnesses by ear

An earlobe creased at a 45 degree angle toward the shoulder may be a warning sign of cardiovascular disease. Reports in the British

Heart Journal and Modern Medicine found that men with ear creases were 55 percent more likely to die of heart disease than men without ear creases. Weight doesn't appear to affect whether or not people have creases in their ears because both thin and fat people have creases in equal numbers. Ear creases were a more accurate predictor of dying suddenly from a heart attack than other risk facts, such as previously diagnosed heart disease. Creased ear lobes are also linked to genetic disorders, such as Beckwith-Wiedemann syndrome

Chapter 5
Eyes

Bloodshot or inflamed eyes can signal everything from an infection to gastroenteritis, or even autoimmune diseases such as arthritis. High cholesterol can cause a white ring around the iris or colored part of the eye, due to fatty deposits, as can small waxy lumps on the skin around the eye. Pale eyelids may indicate anemia. Drooping eyelids, often caused by eyestrain, can also be signs of either a stroke or even lung cancer, which can put pressure on a nerve group in the chest that affects the eyes. Bulging eyes, as per ophthalmologist Marc Werner may be a sign of thyroid disease.

The appearance of the iris of the eye indicates you a lot about your health. (Iridology is science devoted to it) You can, however; look at the colour of the sclera (the whites). If you are tense the small blood vessels will be slightly shriveled. If you have a lot of toxins in the system or you have been stressed for a long period of time, then the shriveled capillaries will have burst. If this has happened recently you will see a reddish colour in the sclera. (Diagram a) That means that fresh blood has seeped out of the blood vessels.
Over a period of time the iron in the blood is converted into ferrous chloride or ferrous oxide, which is brownish red in colour. You could say your eyes have gone rusty (see diagram b). If this has happened you are not 100 per cent healthy.

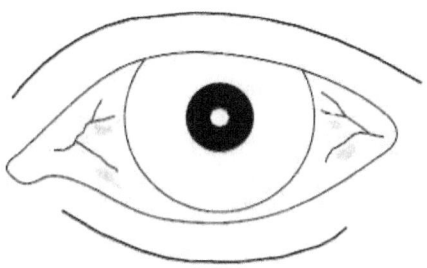

Diagram a
vessels in the sclera (white of the eye)

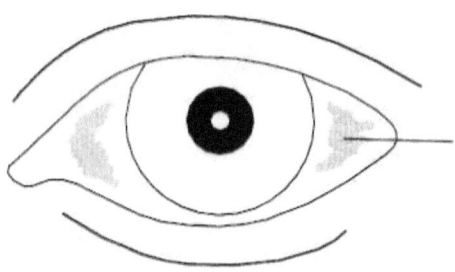

diagram b

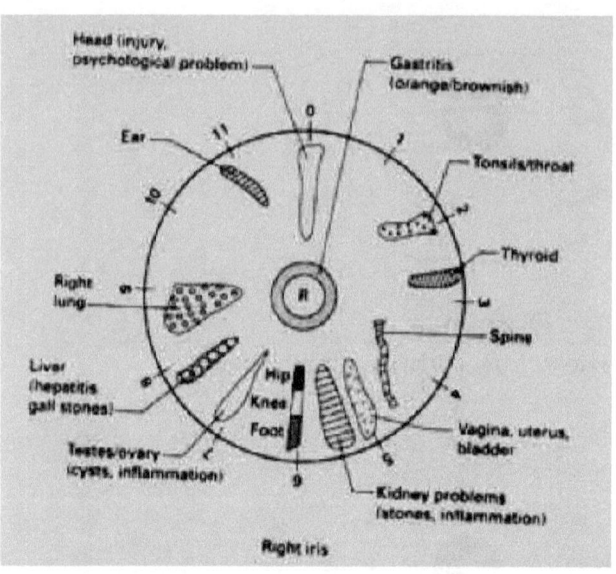

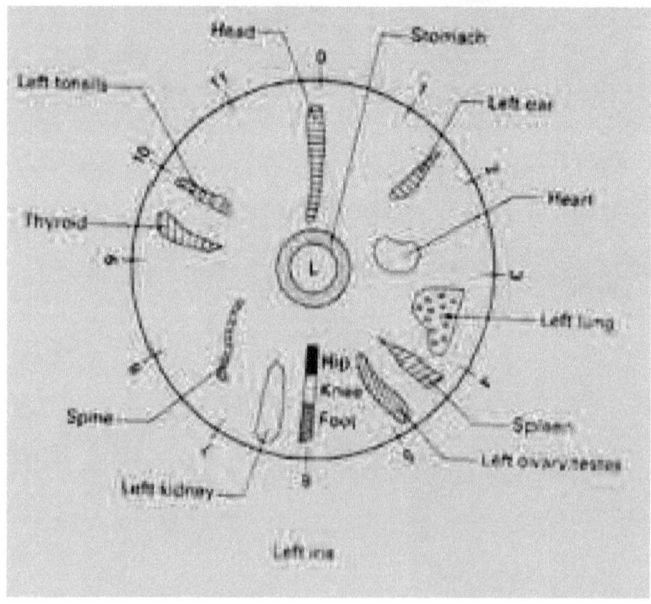

Chapter 6

Other parts of body

Many expert diagnosticians believe our faces reflect our state of health.
They believe that warning signs like bloodshot eyes are all too often ignored as inconsequential when they could in fact be evidence of serious illness. Here are some of the medical problems that a long look in the looking glass can give guidance.

1.Skin

A blotchy or irritated complexion can indicate irritable bowel

syndrome, and polycystic ovary syndrome can cause acne in women

due to hormonal changes. Changes in skin color, especially to yellow,

can be a sign of jaundice and liver problems. A color change to orange

can be a sign of too much beta-carotene from eating too many yellow

and red fruits and vegetables. Sallow skin can be a symptom of

dehydration.

2.Hair

Sudden loss of hair shows either deficiency of minerals or vitamins,

or a restriction of the blood flow to the scalp.

Vitamin B-12 is essential for hair pigmentation, so if you're prematurely going gray, you might be deficient in the vitamin.
This condition is known as pernicious anemia, and

other symptoms can be weight loss, fatigue, and diarrhea.

Low iron levels could cause thinning hair in women, or it can signal a deficiency of vitamin D. In both sexes, thinning hair on the head and/or eyebrows, especially if accompanied by dry skin and fatigue, can be a symptom of an underactive thyroid gland.

3.Nose

A red bulbous nose has long been associated with alcohol causing the blood vessels in the nose to dilate but a red nose can also be caused by illness, chronic sinus problems, and even eating spicy foods. Red noses (and faces) are often a result of rosacea, an adult skin disease in which the blood vessels of the face enlarge and turn the nose red, making the face appear flushed.

4.Mouth

Bleeding gums are commonly a sign of gingivitis due to poor oral hygiene, but they can also indicate leukemia, which affects blood clotting. Minor burns from food can cause ulcers in the mouth, as can even stress, but if they last more than two weeks they need to be evaluated for cancer. Cracked lips, especially at the corners of the mouth and if they're persistent, can be caused either by anemia or diabetes. Pale lips can be a sign of low oxygen levels in the blood caused by heart or lung problems, and also can be yet another indicator or anemia. White patches on the tongue can be caused by a fungus called thrush, and can be cleared quickly by an anti-fungal mouthwash.

White patches that are not sore and don't go away need to be checked for cancerous cell changes.

In fact, any sore or discolored area in your mouth that doesn't heal within two weeks should be investigated by a professional, advises The Oral Cancer Foundation.

5.Weight

If you're not trying to slim down, but suddenly drop 5 percent of your body weight in a month or 10 percent in six months, it's time to call the doctor. Sudden, unexplained weight loss could be a symptom of liver disease or diabetes, says the Mayo Clinic. Also, if you feel full after eating little, a gastrointestinal disorder could be the culprit, or, according to the University of Maryland Medical Center, a problem with your gallbladder. But it could also indicate a more serious condition, such as pancreatic cancer or ovarian cancer.

Chapter 7

SHIATSU AND REFLEXOLOGY

Acupressure is a very good method of diagnosis and cure. This is Chinese and Indian methods of cure. This is based on the principle of energy/ Prana flow. It believes that there is flow of energy in the body and any blockage in the system causes disease. While Chinese call this flow of energy as Chi, Indians call this Prana. Chinese believe that Chi is of two types namely YANG and YIN. Where Yang is positive energy, Yin is negative and a balance must be maintained in flow of these energies to keep good health. It is necessary to understand the Principle of these energies. Indians balance the flow of these energies through Yoga and Pranayama. Indians also believe that energy is focused mostly at seven points known as Chakras. There are 7 Chakras. Each Chakra emits light of different colour and these lights cause Aura. Balance of these Chakras should be maintained. Any decrease in the strength of the lights of Chakras denotes disease connected with that Chakra. Modern doctors and scientists have accepted the concept of Chakras and they call them glands. Any disturbance in the glands can lead to serious diseases. Now there are equipments available to check the Aura and determine the disease due to mal functioning of Chakras.

YANG and YIN complement and balance each other. Even if we don't understand (or believe in) yin and yang, we can see how nature and humans balance their energies in a similar way.
As per Chinese system, there are invisible lines in the

human body called meridians. Body energy is said to flow along these meridians. There are points (called tsubos) on these meridians that are connected with all the systems of our body, both physical and mental.

• Yang meridians flow down the body.
• Yin meridians flow up the body.

A person follows either a yin-type or yang-type pattern of behaviour but no person is completely yang or completely Yin,but an ever changing balance of the two.

Chinese bring in balance of these forces through massaging and pressing of these points and the process is known as SHIATSU.
Other method of treatment is similar to Shiatsu but here the pressure is normally given in hands or feet. This is known as Reflexology.
Reflexology is in widespread use in many parts of the world and is used as a diagnostic tool as well as a treatment. Reflexology has come from the word 'Reflex'. Working of nervous system in the body is through Reflexes. Experience has also shown that unlike nerves, these energy reflexes do not cross over the spinal column and react without going through the spinal connector nerves, following instead the body's zone lines. For example, the eye reflex in the left foot will react from the *left* eye and not the right as might be expected from the study of the central nervous system. Organs which are in the same zone are often related and the related reflex (as well as the affected reflex) may show a blockage, e.g., eyes and kidneys are in the same zone. Success of treatment depends on the skill of the operator.

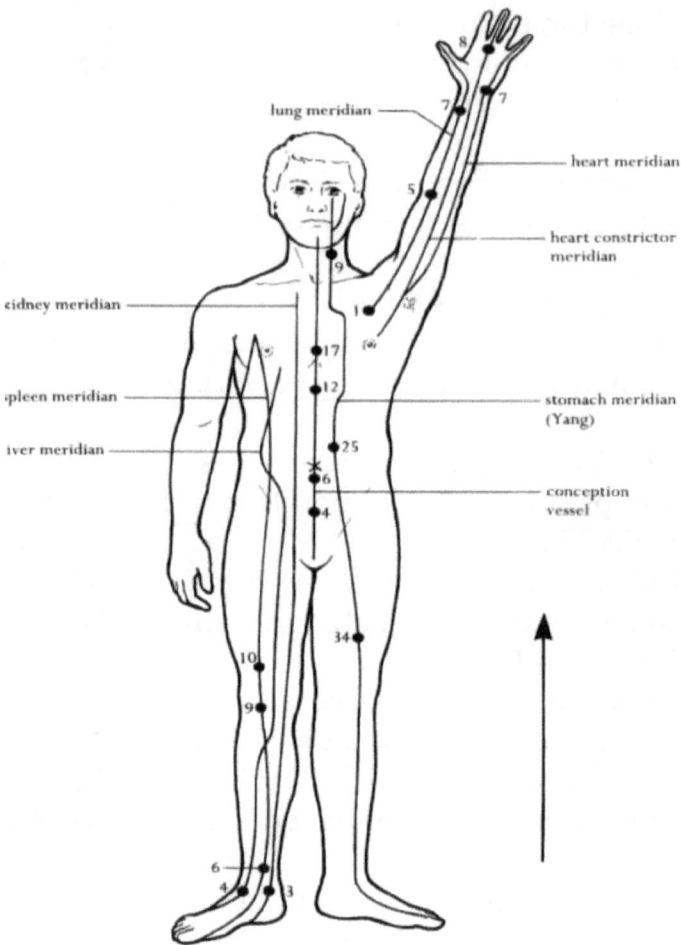

lung meridian

heart meridian

heart constrictor meridian

kidney meridian

spleen meridian

stomach meridian (Yang)

liver meridian

conception vessel

Yin Meridian

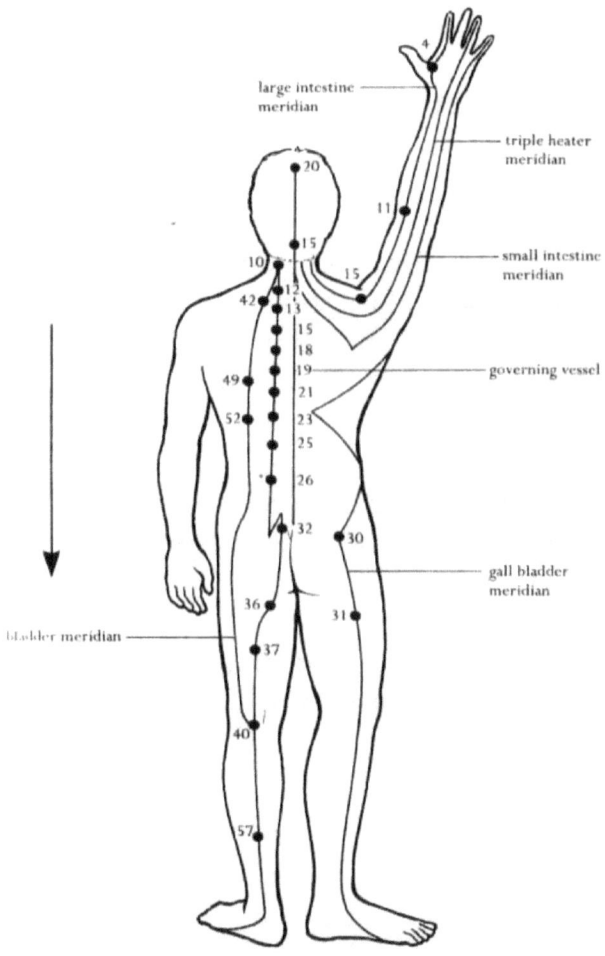

large intestine meridian

triple heater meridian

small intestine meridian

governing vessel

gall bladder meridian

bladder meridian

20

15

10

42

12
13

15

18

19

21

23

25

26

32

30

36

31

37

40

57

49

52

11

15

Yang Meridian

Reflex points are easiest to find in the feet, though they are also found in other extremities of the body, i.e. hands, ears and tongue. Each organ and muscle in the body is connected without crossing the spinal column by an energy pathway to a point in the foot (see Figure) and hand. Pressure on these reflex points indicates the

probable where there may be some disorder
(not the *cause or nature* of the disorder - only that some
 disorder is there) and treatment then given brings about
relaxation, as well as tending to normalize body conditions
out of balance.

The most fascinating thing about these reflex points is
that they come to the surface in exactly the same relative
position as they are found in the body, and are most easily
found on the soles of the feet and hands. If you imagine
that with the feet close together, looking at the soles, the
big toes are the head, the balls of the feet are the shoulders
and down the centre is the spine - the curve of each foot here
is even identical to the view of a person's back. The foot
even narrows around t i n waist area. Thus, all organs
found above the waist in the body are found above the
waist of the foot, those positioned b e low are found below.
This shows that a basic knowledge of body is beneficial
 in reflexology.

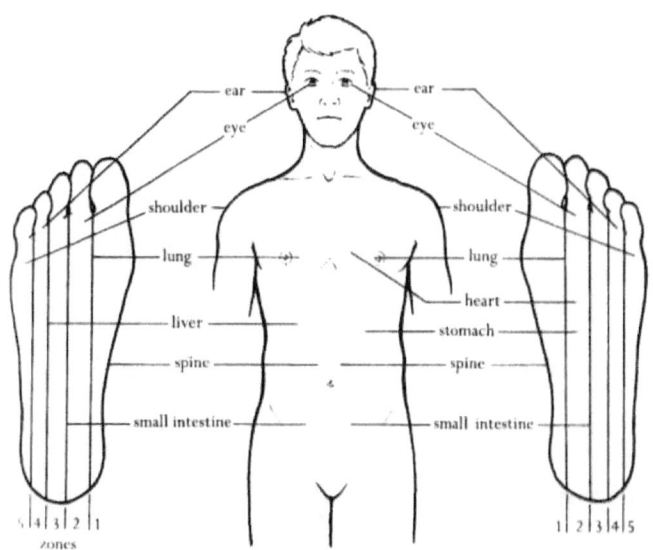

General relationship of body to foot area.

Chapter 8

Hands and Feet: (Reflexology or Zone Therapy

As all the meridians either start from the fingers of hands or end on the fingers of the feet, it is natural that all the parts of the body are connected to the hands or the feet and posterio-Inferior regions or the ankle joints and all points of diagnosis and treatment are found there. To find the problem of the body, it is essential that all points on the feet and hands are scanned thoroughly for tender/painful points. These points should be intermittently pressed for treatment. Press each point for 5 seconds, release for 3 seconds, and repeat for 2/3 minutes, twice or thrice a day. Charts of feet and hands as depicted below should be checked and treatment given as required on the particular points

This system is not only curative but preventive also. Check on the pressure points for five minutes a day and treatment will keep you healthy. It also indicates the incoming ailments and timely treatment saves one from medication and other vagaries of ailments.

For parts and organs of left side of the body, left hand or foot, and for the right side, right hand and or foot should be treated.

However, 5 minutes duration should not be applied on point No.36 (which is the point of Heart); only one minute duration should be applied on this point at a time, totaling 2 minutes in the whole day.

This treatment can be given to oneself and can be given to any other person without any adverse reactions. Even a child can treat oneself. Even while taking medicines under other systems of treatment from Doctors, this therapy can also be taken, as it will help in expediting the cure.

This system also serves as a self-diagnosing method by pressing the points and checkup the Charts From this method it is not only possible to diagnose after the problem has started, but as mentioned earlier the disease that is likely to start can be prevented.

The diagrams nos.21, 22, 23, 24, 25, 26 show how the different parts of the body are connected to the hands and feet.

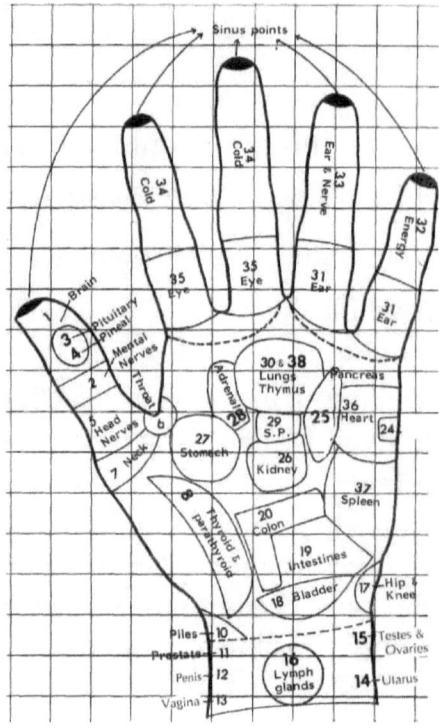

Fig21:Left Hand

Location and Number of points connected with different organs and endocrine glands.

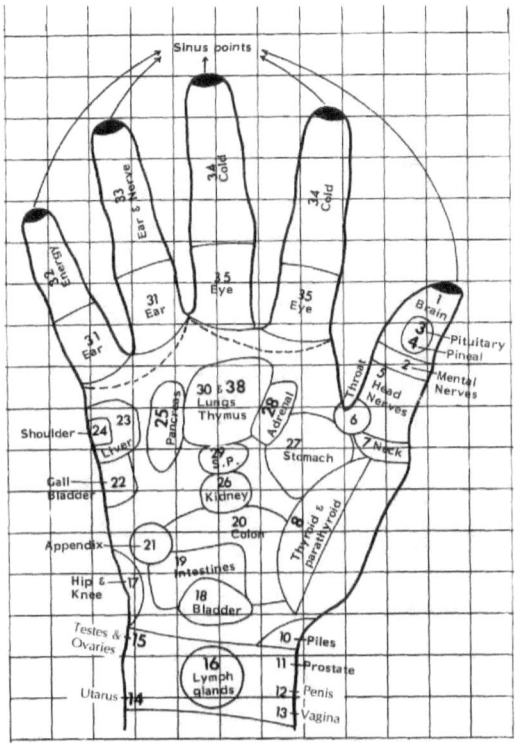

Fig22: Right-Hand

For treatment: Pressure is to be applied
on and around these points of palms and hands

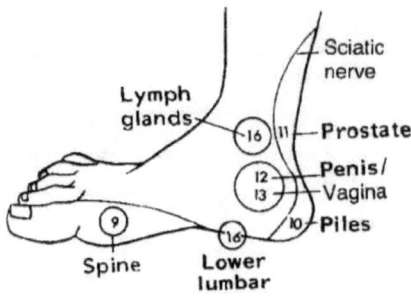

Fig23 inside of foot

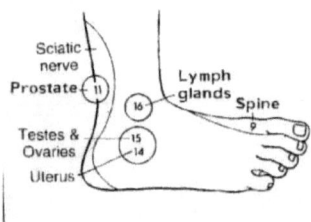

Fig24 outside of foot

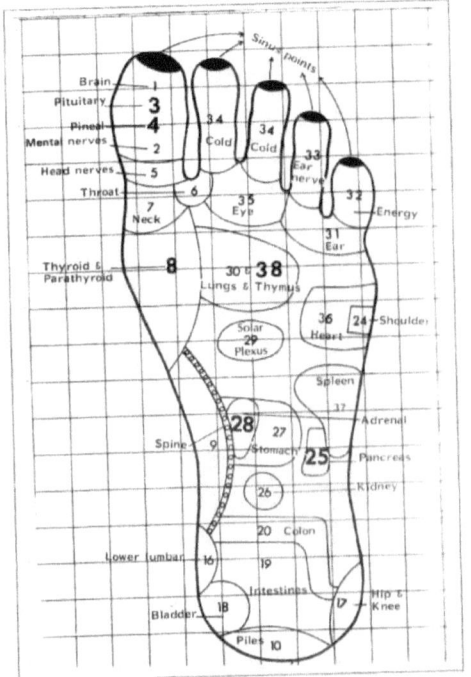

Fig 25 Left Sole

For treatment: Pressure is to be applied
on and around these points of soles

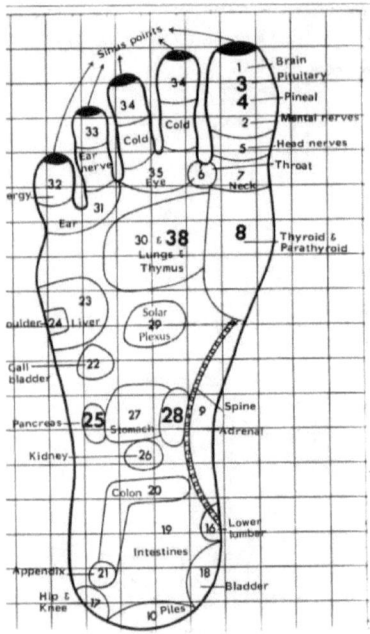

Fig 26 Right Sole

For treatment: Pressure is to be applied
on and around these points of soles

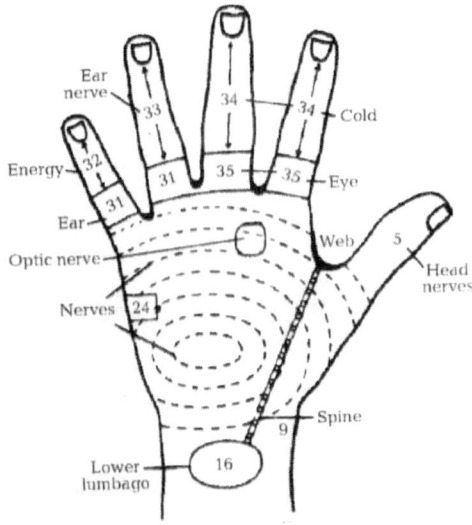

Fig 27 Left Hand back

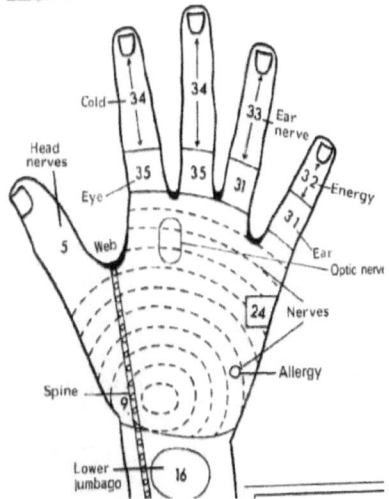

Fig 28 Right Hand back

Point No.	Pressure points , disease
1.	Brain, anemia, cough, mental problem, tonsillitis
2	Mental Nerves, anemia, cough, tonsillitis
3	Pituitary glands, cough, , mental problem, tonsillitis
4	Pineal, cough, tonsillitis
5	Head nerves, cough, tonsillitis
6	Throat, cough, measles, tonsillitis
7	Neck, cough, , measles, tonsillitis
8	Thyroid and parathyroid, , mental problem
9	Spine, back pain
10	Piles
11	Prostrate, bed wetting, leucorrhea, obesity, stone
12	Penis, bed wetting, leucorrhea, obesity, stone
13	Vagina, bed wetting, leucorrhea, obesity , stone
14	Uterus, bed wetting, leucorrhea, obesity, stone
15	Testes and ovaries, bed wetting, leucorrhea

obesity , stone

16	Lymph glands(front) and lower lumbar (back), back pain, boils, leucorrhea, , mental problem
17	Hip and knee
18	Bladder, bed wetting, stone
19	Intestines, diabetes, diahhrea, dysentry, stomach ache
20	Colon, diahhrea, dysentery
21	Appendix (front), allergies (back side)
22	Gall bladder, stomach ache
23	Liver, anemia, diabetes, dysentery, stomach ache
24	Shoulders
25	Pancreas, diabetes, dysentery
26	Kidneys, bed wetting, anemia, boils, diabetes, , mental problem, stone
27	Stomach, diabetes, dysentery, leucorrhea, stomach ache
28	Adrenal
29	SOLAR PLEXUS, stomach ache, measles
30	Lungs, cough, measles

31	Ear, slipped disc (both sides)
32	Energy
33	Nerves of ears
34	Cold, , measles
35	eyes
36	Heart , measles
37	Spleen, anemia, cough, diahhrea, tonsillitis
38	Thymus, measles

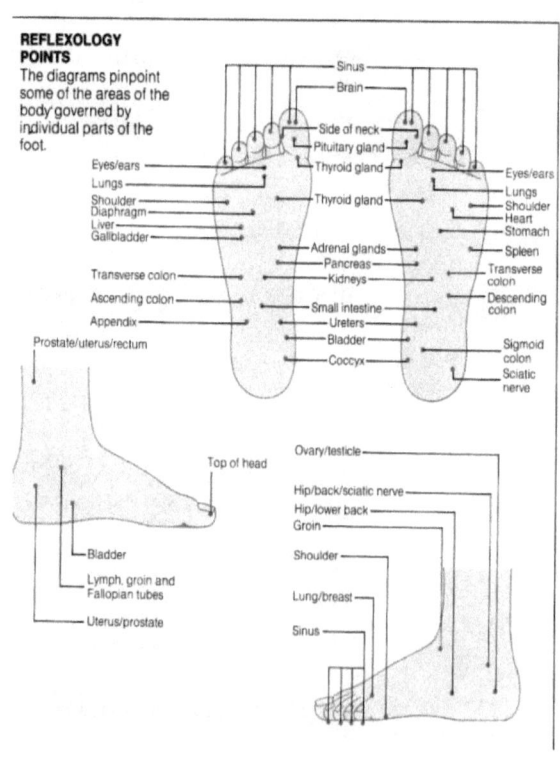

REFLEXOLOGY POINTS
The diagrams pinpoint some of the areas of the body governed by individual parts of the foot.

Rub fingers of both hands. And press the finger tips. Also apply pressures to finger tips of feet also. The islets of Langerhans are in the pancreas and are responsible for the secretion of insulin and glucogen to maintain correct levels of glucose in the blood. When insufficient insulin is produced. glucose levels in the blood rise, resulting in diabetes mellitus.

The adrenal glands lie above the kidneys. They produce two main types of hormone: the outer layer produces steroid hormones that balance the salt, sugar and water concentration in the body, while the inner layer produces the adrenalin necessary to stimulate the `fight or flight' reaction.

Chapter 9

Diagnosis by Pulse Examination

Most people already know that the pulse reflects heart rate, which is normally between 60-90 beats per minute. Whether it is too slow, too fast or irregular, it can indicate a possible heart problem. In western countries medicine recognizes only one type of pulse taken on the radial artery near the wrist to check its rate, rhythm, volume etc. However, according to Traditional Ayurvedic and Chinese Medicine, the pulse reveals more than just heart rate. Chinese pulse diagnosis is an extremely complex subject and an important diagnostic tool. This is why we take pulse readings much longer than you normally experience at a western medical office.

As per Chinese diagnosis inequality of energy in certain meridians is the expression of a pathological condition. Therefore, it is very important to try to locate where the meridians with excess or depletion energy are. In addition, during actual acupressure treatment, improvement can be monitored on the pulses. Though this is a subjective diagnosis, but I have met an acupuncturist who depended on it very accurately and cured most of the disease by acupuncture. I have seen one patient who was completely immobile getting cured by acupuncture. The disease was diagnosed only through pulse checking.

The Normal Pulse: reflects good Heart Qi and Blood. It should be calm, smooth, soft, but not too soft, and not slow, rapid, rough or hard. It should be regular. Its quality should not change very often or easily. Deep level and rear position should be felt clearly, indicating that the Kidneys are healthy. In Ayurveda, the humoral imbalances in three Doshas- Vata, Pitta, and Kapha - can be diagnosed by pulse examination. The Ayurvedic pulse also helps to determine the balance of Prana, tejas and ojas. Ayurvedic pulse measurement is done by placing index, middle and ring finger on the wrist. The index finger is placed below the wrist bone on the thumb side of the hand (radial styloid). This finger represents the Vata dosha. The middle finger and ring finger are placed next to the index finger and represents consequently the Pitta and Kapha doshas of the patient. Pulse can be measured in the superficial, middle, and deep levels thus obtaining more information regarding energy imbalance of the patient.

The Chinese Pulses can be considered as the characteristic diagnostic method. Through feeling the pulses (note the plural) the practitioner assesses the condition of any organ or any part of the body, including psychological states. The pulses technique has been developed over many centuries.

In Traditional Chinese Medicine, pulse diagnosis is important for two reasons - it can give very detailed information on the state of the internal organs and it reflects the whole complex of Qi, Blood Yin, Yang and frankly, every part of the body. It gives the doctor an indication of the overall constitution of a person. Just as the tongue can reflect these phenomena, so does the pulse. Pulse diagnosis is a very subtle skill. We take the pulse on the radial artery, dividing it into three sections on the wrist and detecting it at three different levels. The three wrist sections of the pulse on the radial artery are the front, middle and rear, respectively. The three levels are superficial (pressing lightly), middle (pressing a little deeper) and deep (pressing even deeper). The three levels at each of the three sections on the wrist are referred to as the "Nine Regions."

As is shown in the diagram the pulse is divided into three positions on each wrist. The first pulse closest to the wrist is the *cun* (inch) position, the second *guan* (gate), and the third pulse position furthest away from the wrist is the *chi* (foot). Each position represents a pair of organs, with different organs apparent on the superficial, middle, and deep level. Various classic texts cite different pairings of organs, some omitting the second organ from the pulse entirely. Generally, the first position on the left hand represents the heart and small intestine, the second, liver and gallbladder, and third the kidney yin and the bladder. On the right hand, the first position is representative of the lungs and large intestine, the second of the spleen and stomach, and the third represents the kidney yang and uterus or triple burner. The strengths and weaknesses of the positions are used to assess the patient diagnostically, along with the different qualities and speed of the pulse. The photograph illustrations show how the fingers should be placed in order to take the pulses. Before taking the pulses the patient should be recumbent, relaxed and quiet. Pulses on the right wrist are felt with the fingers of the right hand; pulses on the left wrist are taken with the fingers of the left. These pulses are felt on both radial arteries with three fingers next to each other and, at the same time, in two different pressure strengths (each pulse extending for approximately half an inch). Thus, the state of six different organs is to be ascertained under the three fingers on the radial pulse on each side, i.e., the state of 12 different organs. The exact positions are found by first placing the middle finger on the middle of the apophasis of the radius, the first and ring fingers then fall naturally into the correct positions. The first finger will be in the small hollow on the proximal side of the apophasis; and the ring finger at the base of the thumb, just proximal to the thenar eminence (see diagram). The pulse is felt with the pad of the finger (last phalange) lightly rested in position for the superficial pulse; and pressed heavily for the deep pulse, not so heavily, of course, as to crush the artery against the bone. On the right wrist where the pulse is taken at three levels, the pressure must be delicately adjusted to light, medium, and heavy pressure. The practitioner by checking the pulses actually measures their condition (strengths YIN/ YAN). Treatment at Points can be either in tonification or in sedation (dispersion). If there is not enough activity or tone the condition is said to be YIN, and stimulation (tonification) is required. If there is too much activity (hyper tonicity) the condition is said to be YAN and sedation (dispersion) action must be taken to restore the balance.

In healthy persons the vital *(Yang-Yin)* force flows smoothly, freely throughout the body in dynamic equilibrium. All sickness, slight or serious, is derailment of YANG-YIN equilibrium. The treatment, therefore, is directed towards the restoration of normal YANG-YIN balance.

Chinese practitioner not only does the treatment of, but also *foresees* the probable long-term consequences of present YANG-YIN imbalance if left untreated. The Chinese practitioner anticipates and treats a disease before it happens; thus preventing it from ever happening.

The practitioner represents the state of the pulse by assigning a number from 0 to 8. 4 represents Normal, 3 to 0 represents a YIN condition, 5 to 8 represents a YANG condition. Any departure from normal (4) indicates that the organ associated with that pulse is deranged or troubled to *some degree* and requires treatment either in tonification or in sedation. According to Dr. de la Fuye, a relatively little experience suffices to enable one to recognize a YIN or a YANG condition, but it takes a long experience to be able to form a clear picture of the illness and to assess the exact points to be treated.

Dr. Stiefvater's simplification of pulse interpretation should, however, enable a practitioner to make a sound beginning in the general assessment of YIN or YANG conditions of Yin and yang organs. Thus, by examining the strength and quality of the pulse at these three levels, we get a better idea of the pathology of Qi, Blood and Yin, and of the relative state of Yin and Yang

Small, thin, fine:	Insufficiency.
Full and hard:	Hypertension,Hyperfunction.
Soft and strong:	Inflammation.
Small, hard and pointed:	Spasticity, contractures, usually an organ painful.
Overflowing and large:	Excess, usually with inflammation and pain

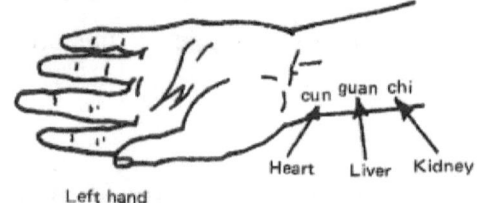

Left hand

LEFT WRIST

FRONT: HEART / SMALL INTESTINE
MIDDLE: LIVER / GALL BLADDER
REAR: KIDNEY / BLADDER

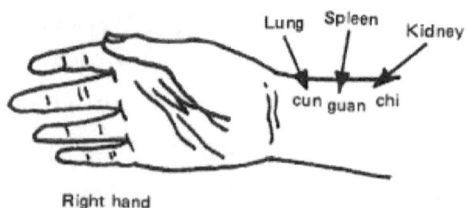

Right hand

RIGHT WRIST

FRONT: LUNGS / LARGE INTESTINE
MIDDLE: SPLEEN / STOMACH
REAR: GATE OF **Vitality** FIRE

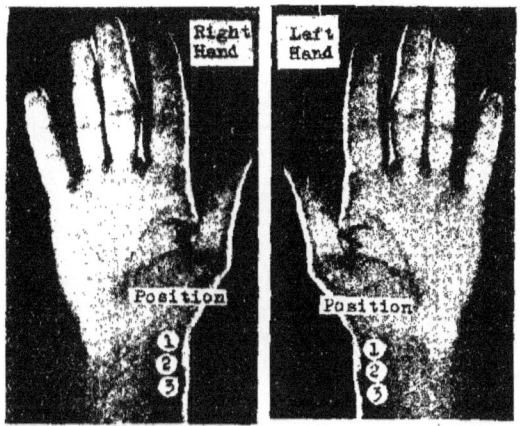

Position showing placement of fingers for taking pulses

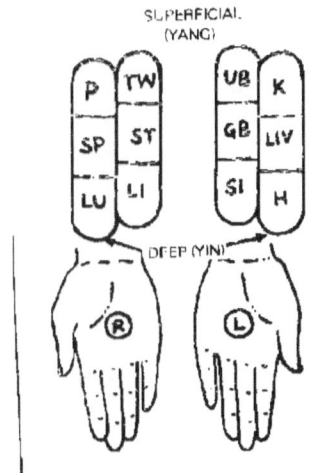

Relation of pulses with parts of body

On the right wrist	On the left wrist
Deep superficial	Superficial Deep
Pericardium Triple warmer	Urinary Bladder Kidney
Spleen Stomach	Gall bladder Liver
Lung Large intestine	Small intestine Heart

Chapter 10

Reiki

Reiki is a simple, natural and safe method of spiritual healing and self-improvement that everyone can use. It has been effective in helping virtually every known illness as it reunites the trinity of Mind, Body and Spirit. It also works in conjunction with all other medical or therapeutic techniques to relieve side effects and promote recovery

Reiki is derived from two Japanese words. Rei means universal, spirit power and gives supernatural knowledge or spiritual consciousness.
Ki or Chi means life force energy. Ki means the same as Chi in Chinese, Prana in Sanskrit. It is the vital life force or the universal life force. This nonphysical energy animates all living things and is used by all healers. As long as something is alive, it has life force/Pranas circulating through it and surrounding it; when it dies, the life force departs. The Chinese and Indians place great importance on this life force. It is used in meditative breathing exercises called Pranayam. This energy in modern world is cosmic energy.

Thus Reiki means the Power to transmit and receive universal life force energy.

If your life force (Ki) is low, or if there is a restriction in its flow, you will be more vulnerable to illness or feel stress. When it is high and flowing freely, you are more capable of being happy and healthy.

Life force plays an important role in everything we do. The ability to use Reiki is not taught in the usual sense, but is transferred to the student during a Reiki class. This ability is passed on during an "attunement" given by a Reiki master and allows the student to tap into an unlimited supply of "life force energy." It balances the chakras/glands and thus improves one's and other's health. Learning Reiki is a simple technique.

As Reiki is cosmic energy it helps us in diagnosis and cure of many diseases. The person who is not attuned can learn the method of diagnosis easily. He should rub both his hands vigorously for about 2 minutes, then he should pull both the hands facing each other about a foot and again bring near at a distance of 1 to 2 inches and again pull back to distance of one foot and back to 1 to 2 inches. He should repeat this process about 6 to 7 times. He will feel vibrations in the hands. Now he should scan his whole body with hands keeping on each part of body for at least 3 minutes. He will feel either vibration in his hands or feel the diseased body to be hot or cold. This method can not only be used for diagnosis but for treatment.

Conclusion

Diagnosis through self-inspection has scientific roots and can be learnt with little efforts. This can help to diagnose the diseases and take action in time and save suffering and money as actions can be taken to prevent and cure diseases in time without allowing it to aggravate. These methods are now widely accepted not only in India and China but throughout the world. MedlinePlus- Web site of the National Institutes of Health of USA (Produced by the National Library of Medicine) also gives some details of these diagnostic procedures.

www.ingramcontent.com/pod-product-compliance
Lightning Source LLC
Chambersburg PA
CBHW050502290526
45786CB00006B/2395